# Homemade Lotions

## 40 Organic Recipes

Table of Contents

## Introduction

Human beings have been using beauty products since a very long time. Therefore, in order to moisturize their skin, they employ the use of lotions and sunscreens. These lotions are not only made commercially, but also, a large number of people made the similar products at home. Although, the commercial lotions can be efficacious in the beginning, yet they possess various toxin chemicals, which can hamper the skin cells. Considering this problem, the importance of homemade products seems inevitable. Therefore, this book is designed to provide efficient lotion recipes, which can be created at home.

This book covers numerous kinds of recipes to improve the skin. To begin, the recipes for homemade lotions for oil skin are included. Furthermore, the recipes which are used to make organic lotions for dry skin are discussed. In addition to that, the recipes for men lotion are elaborated. Moreover, the recipes which help you in making lotions for neutral skin are also incorporated in the book. Finally, the recipes, which help in the creation of butter based lotions are encompassed.

Therefore, this book is an amazing manual to make homemade lotions. The lotions created using these recipes will help you in improving your skin. Moreover, they do not possess harmful chemicals which can cause numerous problems. It is because of the efficiency of the homemade lotions that they are used ubiquitously in various parts of the world. Thus, in order to improve your skin, you must start using the homemade lotions right now. Further, the recipes included here will guide you to begin making and using non-toxic and skin friendly lotions.

# Chapter 1 – Organic Lotion Recipes for Oily Skin

Numerous individuals who have a sleek appearance have a tendency to stay away from creams. The truth of the matter is that sleek skin has a tendency to get dried out; therefore, one must apply no less than a little measure of cream twice in a day. Given underneath are some of the strategies that will help you make a characteristic cream for slick skin.

## 1. Milk and olive oil lotion:

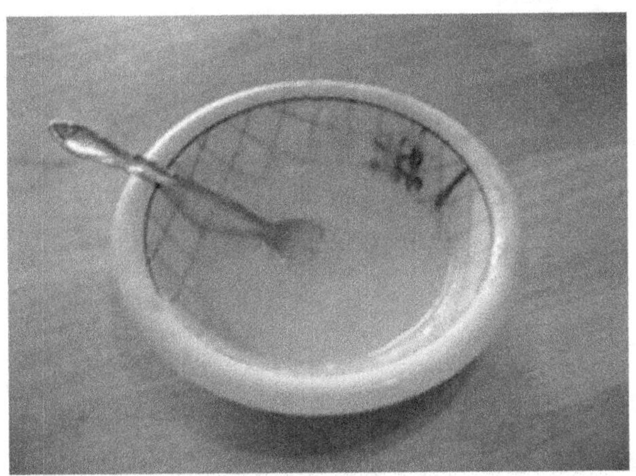

**Ingredients:**

i.    Milk.

ii.   Olive oil.

iii.  Mixing jar.

iv.   Lime juice.

**Methods:**

i.     To begin, take a jar and add one quarter cup milk in it.

ii.     Afterwards, add two tablespoons of olive oil and whisk them together.

iii.     Lastly, include 3 tablespoons of lime juice in the jar and combine them together.

iv.     Now, your moisturizer is ready to be used.

**Advantages of the lotion:**

This lotion holds various advantageous ingredients. The lime juice included in the lotion helps in killing the dead cells. Moreover, the blemishes and acne are also cleansed because of the lime juice. Moreover, olive oil maintains the health of your skin. Further, the lactic acid is used for the softening of your skin.

## 2. Rose petal moisturizer:

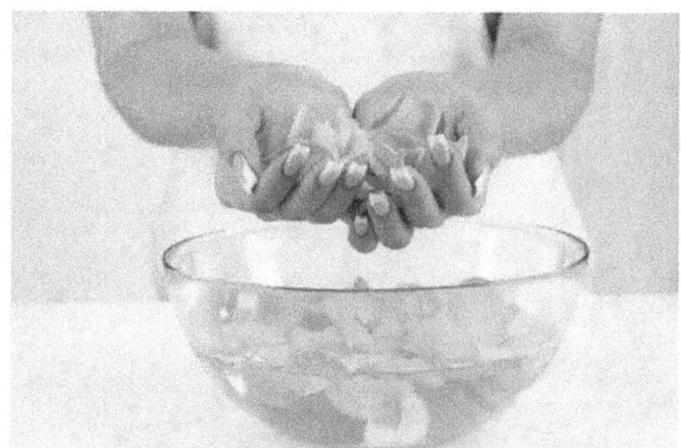

**Ingredients:**

i.      Rose petals.

ii.     Aloe vera juice.

iii.    Rose water.


**Methods:**

i.      To begin, include rose petals in some drops of rose water and boil them together.

ii.     Now, you must filter it as you require liquid mixture.

iii.    Afterwards, once you have cooled the mixture, include almost two tablespoons of aloe juice.

iv.     Cool the mixture in a fridge and apply on your face.


**Advantages of rose petal moisturizer:**

Rose petals moisturizer is amazing because it possess efficacious ingredients. Rose water is used to remove dirt as well as other harmful elements from the skin. Moreover, they refresh your skin. The aloe gel used helps in moisturizing the skin and giving it a fresh look.

3. **Aloe Vera and rose moisturizer:**

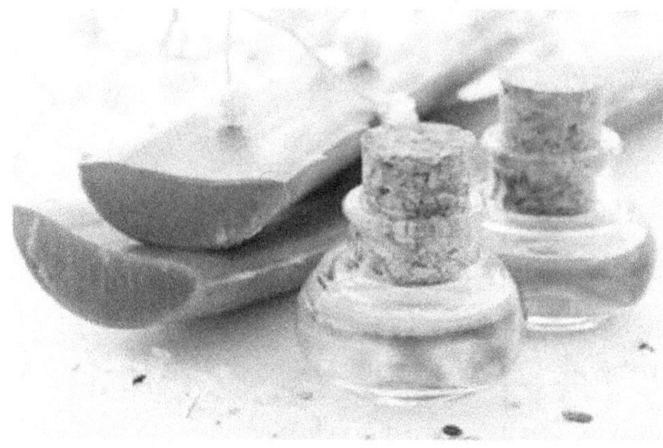

## Ingredients:

i.      Carnauba wax- 2 tablespoons

ii.     Rose oil.

iii.    Water- 2 tablespoons.

iv.     Mixing jar.

v.      Aloe Vera.

vi.     Glass bowl.

vii.    Jojoba oil.


## Methods:

i.      To begin, combine carnauba wax in a jar and six tablespoons of the jojoba oil. Whisk them together.

ii.     Now, add 2 tablespoons of water and stir them well.

iii.    Afterwards, take the jar and put it above boiling water. This will eventually melt the mixture.

iv.    After melting, remove the mixture from heat and cool.

v.    Further, include 2 teaspoons of aloe gel and two drops of rose oil.

vi.    Mix everything together, your lotion is ready.


**Advantages of rose aloe lotion:**

This cream is extremely efficient. It contains jojoba oil, which is used to cleanse the skin. Moreover, the anti-oxidizing property of jojoba oil is used to moisturize the dead skin. In addition, aloe gel is also used for clearing the skin. In addition, carnauba wax also softens your skin.


## 4. Coconut- aloe lotion:

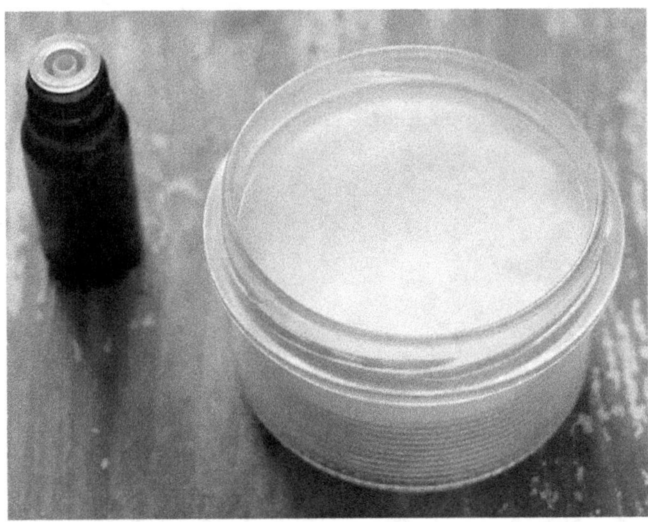

**Ingredients:**

i.      Aloe vera juice- 2 tablespoons.

ii.     Coconut oil- 1/2 cup.

iii.    Essential oils- 10 drops.

iv.     Shea butter- 1/4 cup.

v.      Jojoba oil- 2 tablespoons.

vi.     Cocoa butter- 1/4 cup.

**Method:**

i.      Heat the coconut oil, shea spread and the cocoa margarine over low warmth until dissolved.

ii.     Expel from warmth.

iii.    Include the aloe vera juice, oils and the fluid oil. Now mix to consolidate well.

iv.     Store in holder of your decision. Utilize little canning jugs.

## 5. Vitamin E- almond oil lotion:

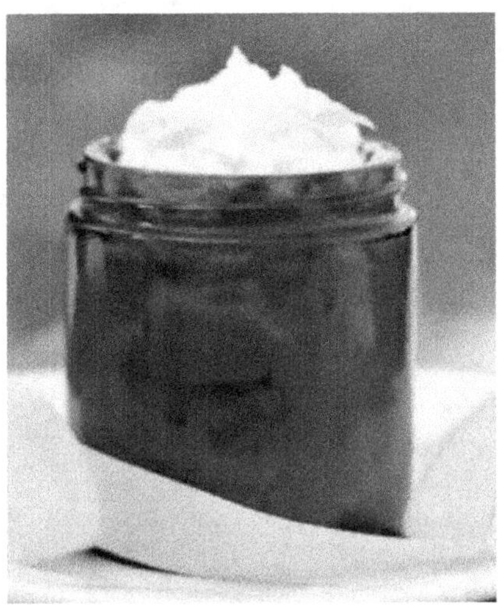

### Ingredients:

i.      Aloe vera gel- 1/2 cup.

ii.     Grated beeswax- 1/4 cup.

iii.    Sweet almond oil- 1 cup.

iv.    Vitamin E oil. 2 teaspoons.

v.     Essential oil- 30 drops.

### Method:

i.      In a medium-sized dish consolidate Vitamin E oil, aloe vera gel, and vital oils. Put aside for some other time, permitting it to come to room temp.

ii.     Add ground beeswax and oil to a glass measuring container. Place measuring glass in a little pot of water and convey water to a delicate bubble. Heat, blending every so often, until beeswax is totally softened then precisely expel measuring container from pot.

iii.    Empty beeswax mixture and put it into blender and permit to cool.

iv.     Once cooled, turn blender on Low. Expel top of blender and pour aloe vera blend in a SLOW, constant stream.

v.      Stop blender as regularly as expected to run a spatula around sides to fuse fixings. On the off chance that fluid is pooling at the top, stop much of the time to push it around with spatula.

vi.     Exchange lotion to clean jugs and refrigerate any part that won't be spent inside a couple of weeks.

**6. Herbal tea-avocado oil lotion:**

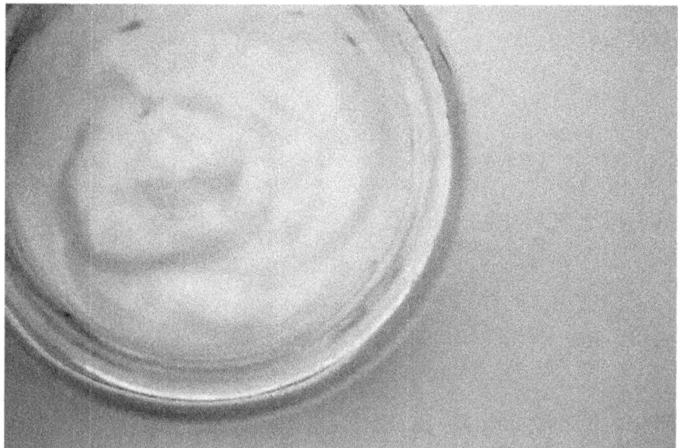

**Ingredients:**

i.      Herbal tea- 1 1/2 cup.

ii.     Avocado oil- 1 1/2 cup.

iii.    Essential oil.

iv.     Beeswax- 6 tablespoons.

**Method:**

i.      Heat the beeswax in a saucepan.

ii.     Then add herbal tea in it and cook for a while.

iii.    Add your oils.

iv.     Cool the mixture, your lotion is ready.

v.

**7.  Cooling aloe- mint body lotion:**

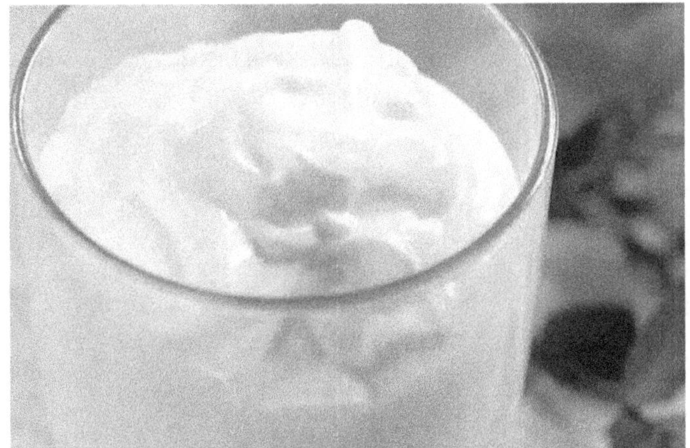

**Ingredients:**

i.      Aloe vera gel- 1 cup.

ii.     Grated beeswax- 1/2 cup.

iii.    Peppermint oil- 1/4 teaspoon.

iv.     Coconut oil- 1 cup.

**Method:**

i.      Put coconut oil and beeswax in a pot over low warmth. Warm just until simply dissolved. Attempt to keep the temperature as low as could be expected under the circumstances to protect the advantages of the coconut oil.

ii.     Expel from the warmth and hand race in the aloe vera gel and peppermint vital oil until it's completely consolidated. You can likewise put the blend over an ice shower and mix the blend with a spatula until it thickens and gets to be velvety white.

iii.    Give the cream a chance to cool to room temperature, for an hour. Whisk once more, or spot in the blender and mix at a medium pace for around half a minute for a fluffier variant.

8. **Homemade non-greasy moisturizing lotion:**

**Ingredients:**

i.      Shea butter- 1 cup.

ii.     Almond oil- 4 tablespoon.

iii.    Lavender oil- 30 drops.


**Method:**

i.      Melt the shea butter and the oils together.

ii.     Put the bowl in the fridge to cool for about 20 minutes, just to the point that the mixture starts to solidify and become translucent.

iii.    Using a handheld mixer, mix until it becomes creamy.

iv.     Transfer to a small jar.

## Chapter 2 – Natural Homemade Lotions for Dry Skin

Dry skin demands extra care as well as oil. Therefore, the recipes used for these lotions must contain some special ingredients. Some of the useful recipes are given in the following text:

### 9. Orange lotion bars:

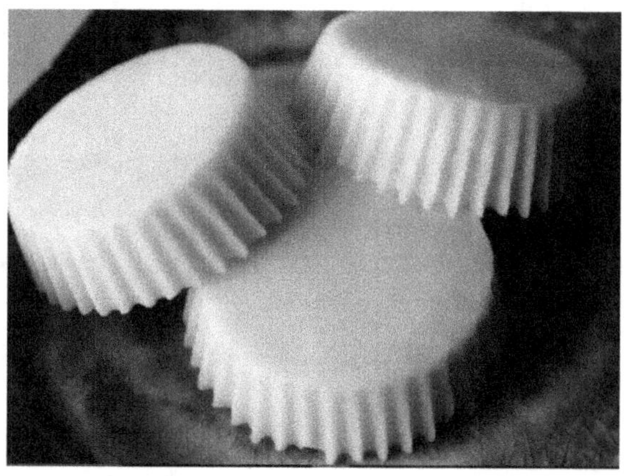

**Ingredients:**

i.      Raw honey.

ii.     Beeswax,

iii.    Shea butter.

iv.    Organic coconut oil.

v.     Olive oil.

vi.    Orange essential oil.

**Method:**

i.  In a twofold heater, liquefy together shea margarine, the beeswax, and coconut oil until they turn into a smooth, uniform fluid.

ii.  Turn the warmth off and include the olive oil, nectar, and vital oil drops.

iii.  In a biscuit tin lined with five cupcake liners, scoop the blend uniformly between the lined cupcake wells.

iv.  Permit to set.

**10.  Moisturizing lotion:**

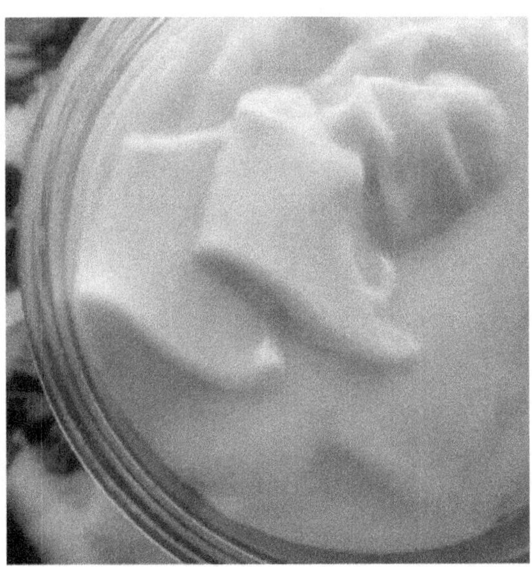

### Ingredients:

i.      Herb oil.

ii.     Kokum spread.

iii.    Any liquid.

iv.     Honey.

v.      Emulsifying wax.

vi.     Citrus extract.


### Method:

i.      In a little sauce skillet, join the herb oil, kokum spread, fluid of decision, nectar, stearic corrosive, emulsifying wax, and citrus extract.

ii.     Heat blend on the stove over low warmth, until the blend is very much joined and totally liquefied. Mix much of the time.

iii.    Expel from stove.

iv.     Utilizing a drenching blender, mix discontinuously until cool, smooth, and thick.

v.      Include rosemary cell reinforcement and fundamental oils.

vi.     Blend well.

vii.    Fill stockpiling jugs.

## 11. Aloe homemade lotion:

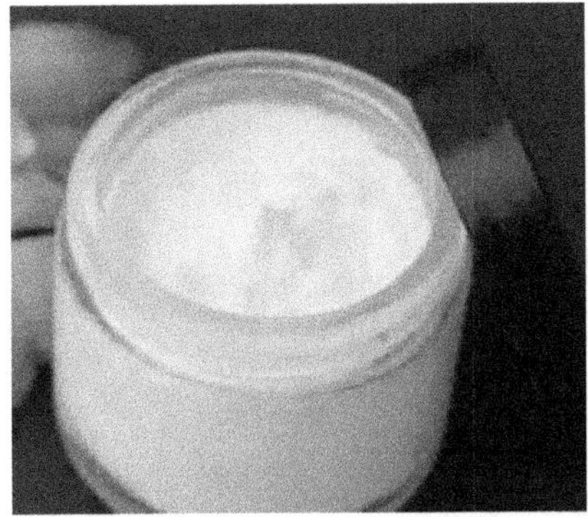

### Ingredients:

i.      Shea butter.

ii.     Jojoba oil.

iii.    Aloe Leaf Juice.

iv.     Vitamin E oil.

v.      Lavender essential oil.

vi.     A pint sized mason jar.

### Method:

i.      Include the Shea spread and Jojoba oil in a container.

ii.     Place a pot on the stove and add some water to it-turn on the warmth to medium high.

iii.    Place the bricklayer container in the pot and mix gradually liquefying the Shea spread with the jojoba oil.

iv.     Once the Shea margarine and jojoba oil is totally dissolved add the aloe juice to the container

v.      With a hand held submersion blender or nourishment processor. Whip the item for no less than 2-3 minutes.

vi.     Include your crucial oil and fill a little jug.


## 12. Calendula cream:

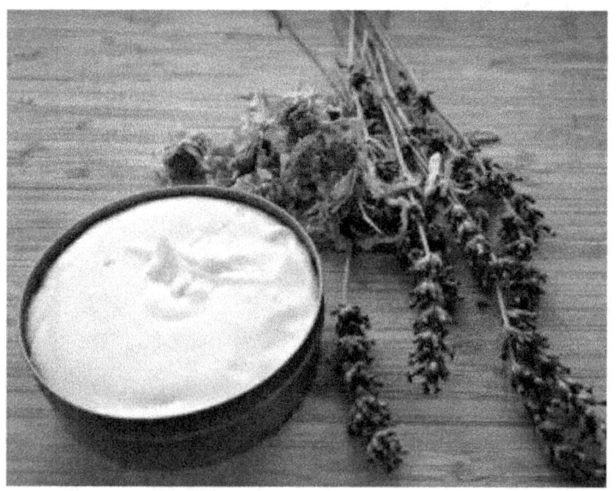

### Ingredients:

i.      Calendula infused oil

ii.     Beeswax.

iii.    Essential oils of your choice.

iv.     Tepid water.

v.      Jars or tins.

**Method:**

i.       Melt the beeswax in the beginning.

ii.       Now add the oils, tepid water in the blender and combine them altogether.

iii.       Let the cream settle before use.

## 13. Hard lotion bars:

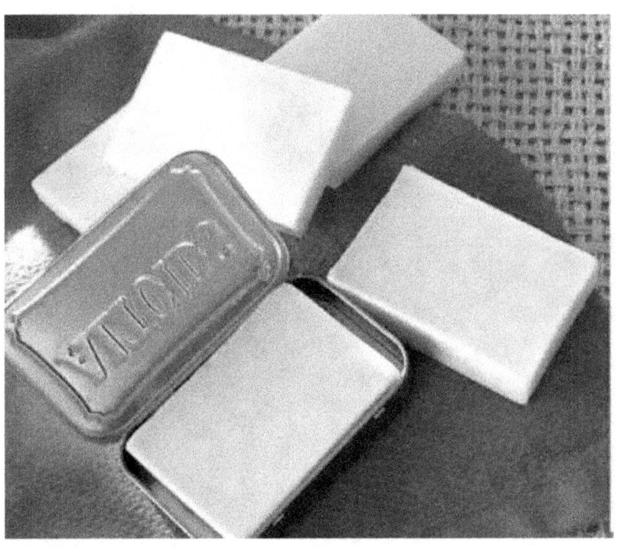

**Ingredients:**

i.       Cocoa Butter.

ii.       Oil e.g. coconut oil.

iii.       Beeswax.

**Method:**

i. Firstly, begin by melting the beeswax and cocoa butter together.

ii. Then melt the coconut oil and combine them together.

iii. Add your essential oil, whisk.

iv. Now let them solidify.

# Chapter 3 – Homemade Lotions for Neutral Skin

Neutral skin possesses a key advantage that it can use various types of lotions. Moreover, these lotions do not even have any hampering effect on the ideal skin. The recipes for some of the lotions that can be used on a neutral skin are as follows:

**14.Homemade scented lotion:**

**Ingredients:**

i.      Unscented lotion.

ii.     A fragrance or oil.

**Method:**

i.      Combine the unscented lotion with a fragrance. Whisk them together.

ii.     You might as well add oil suiting your skin.

**15.Sweet almond lotion:**

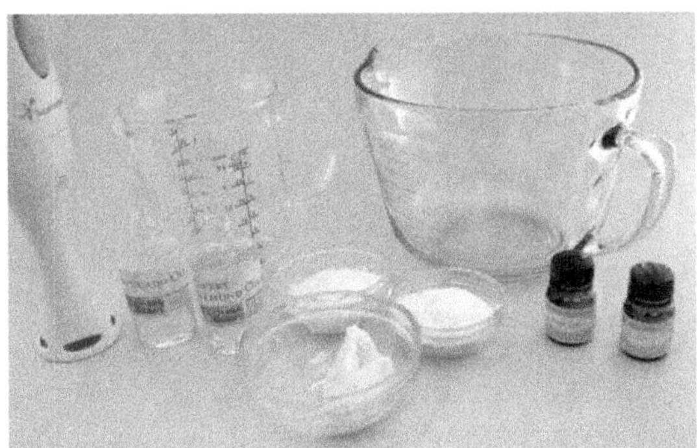

**Ingredients:**

i. Emulsifying Wax.

ii. Distilled Water.

iii. Fragrance.

iv. Shea Butter.

v. Phenonip.

vi. Sweet Almond Oil.

vii. Stearic Acid

viii. Avocado Oil.

**Method:**

i. Firstly, combine emulsifying wax, sweet almond oil, stearic acid and avocado oil altogether and heat it.

ii. Now include shea butter in the mixture and further stir them.

iii. Now include slightly hot distilled water in them.

iv. Whisk, add your special fragrances and your lotion is ready.

## 16. Special tinted moisturizer:

**Ingredients:**

i. Coconut oil.

ii. Homemade powdered foundation.

iii. Vitamin E oil.

iv. Lavender essential oil.

**Method:**

i.  In a little glass dish, melt coconut oil in the microwave or over a twofold evaporator.

ii.  Include homemade powdered establishment, contingent upon how dull you need the tinted cream to be.

iii.  Embed the oil contingent on your skin sort.

## 17. Oatmeal honey lotion:

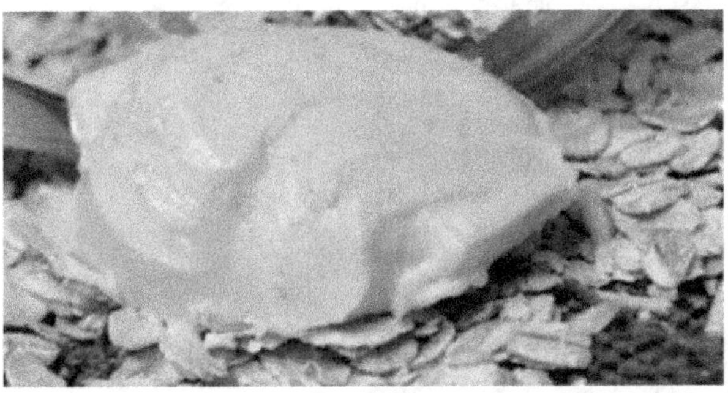

**Ingredients:**

i.  Oatmeal.

ii.  Emulsifying wax.

iii.  Citric acid.

iv.  Cocoa butter

v.  Honey.

vi.  Hazelnut oil.

vii.  Milk.

viii.  Water.

**Method:**

i. Absorb the cereal the water overnight. Mix in the nourishment processor until smooth.

ii. Heat the milk in a pot. Expel from stove and exchange it to a glass jug.

iii. In various pots, over medium low temperature dissolve the cocoa spread, wax and nectar.

iv. Pour the dissolved oil blend gradually into the glass container with milk and water, mixing continually until the two blends are joined. Include the citrus extract. Include mixed oats and blend. The blend will turn out to be smoother while chilling off.

**18.Mint and green tea body lotion:**

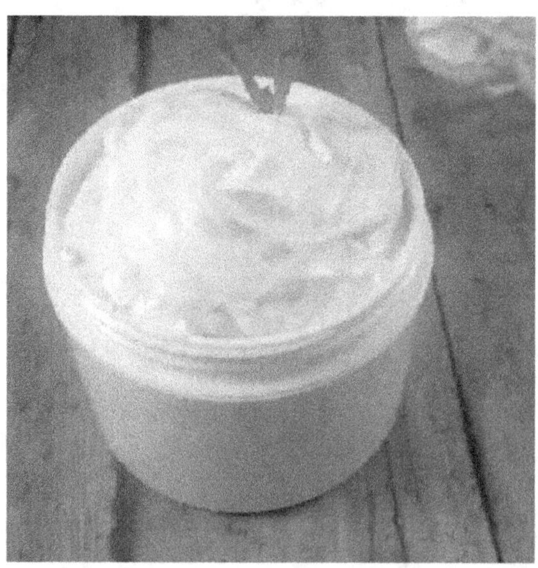

**Ingredients:**

i.      Raw Shea Butter.

ii.     Peppermint Essential oil

iii.    Coconut Oil.

iv.    Fresh Mint Leaves.

v.     Olive oil.

vi.    Macha Powder.

vii.   Vitamin E.

**Method:**

i.      Begin by liquefying the coconut oil and shea spread. Include the olive oil. Empty this oil blend into a blending dish and place in fridge.

ii.     Chill until the majority of your oils begin getting murky. Place your blending dish on the stand blender and join the whip. Whip on rapid until it takes after frothy egg whites.

iii.    Disconnect from blender and spot back in the refrigerator until it is stronger.

iv.    Pour the oils and whip again for 1 moment and after that swing up to rapid and whip for 3 minutes. It ought to begin to look like cream at this point.

v.     Include your mint, macha powder and vitamin E.

vi.    Keep whipping till cushy.

### 19. Crockpot lotion:

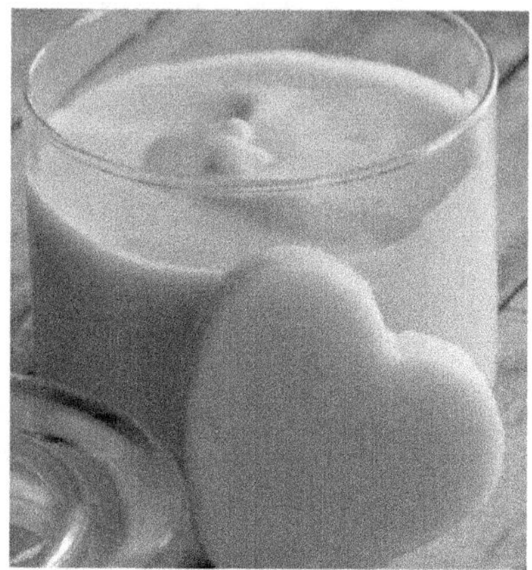

### Ingredients:

i.      Beeswax Pellets.

ii.     Lavender Essential Oil.

iii.    Coconut Oil.

iv.     Vitamin E Oil.

v.      Shea Butter.

### Method:

i.      Firstly, mix butter, beeswax, Vitamin E oil and coconut oil and melt them.

ii.     Now you can fill a mold and make cream bars, or fill a dish and permit to cool for some time.

iii.    Once the Lotion blend is cooled, include the essential Oil and beat on high speeds with a blender.

iv.     This will keep the salve from solidifying, and then you can store it in a sealed shut compartment.


**20.     Anti-wrinkle cream:**

**Ingredients:**

i.      Avocado oil.

ii.     Aloe vera gel.

**Method:**

i.      Join fixings in a glass jug and shake to mix. Touch some on your fingers and back rub into your skin.


**21. Homemade body lotion:**

**Ingredients:**

i.      Baby lotion.

ii.     Scented oils.

iii.    Vaseline.

iv.     Vitamin E cream.

v.      Jars.

**Method:**

i.      Put all fixings into an expansive blending dish and blend until they are frigid.

ii.     Put into holders and appreciate.

22. **Easy beeswax lotion:**

**Ingredients:**

i.      Olive oil.

ii.     Essential oil.

iii.    Coconut oil.

iv.     Beeswax.

v.      Vitamin E oil.

**Method:**

i.      Add coconut oil, beeswax and olive oil in a saucepan.

ii.     Heat them and add then add other oils.

iii.    Combine them together.


23. **Shimmery lotion:**

**Ingredients:**

i.      Lotion.

ii.     Shimmer.

iii.    Jar.

**Method:**

i.      Include shimmer in your favorite lotion.

ii.     Add an essential oil and heat them together with whisking.

iii.    Your lotion is ready.

# Chapter 4 – Homemade Lotions for Men

Lotions are not only used by women, but also, a large number of men use these lotions in order to smooth their skin. Therefore, we have included some of the recipes here to facilitate the male readers.

**24.        Male face moisturizer:**

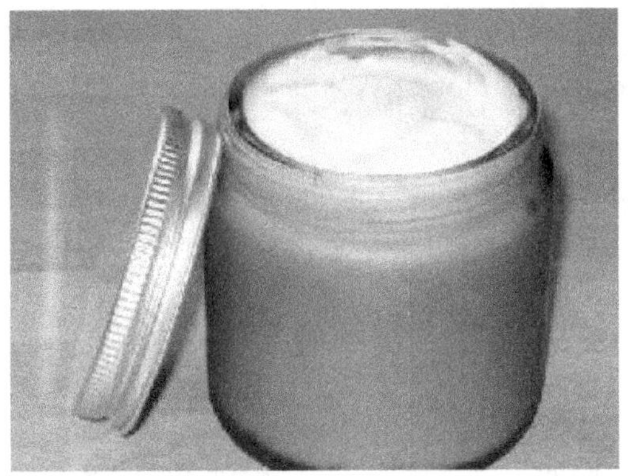

**Ingredients:**

i.      Beeswax- 10 grams.

ii.     Rosehip Seed Oil- 10ml.

iii.    Sweet Almond Oil- 20ml.

iv.    Clary Sage essential oil- 5 drops.

v.     Cedar wood essential oil- 2 drops.

vi.    Bay essential oil- 1 drop.

vii.   Boiling water- 150ml.

**Method:**

i.    With the blossoms and bubbling water, make a home grown mixture. A home grown mixture is made by setting the blooms into a container and pouring bubbling water over them, then cover and leave to cool.

ii.    When cool, strain and put aside prepared for use.

iii.    In the substantial based stainless steel dish, liquefy the beeswax, then beat in the oils as yet beating gradually include the home grown mixture.

iv.    Expel the skillet from the warmth and continue mixing until it has cooled to body temperature.

v.    Blend in the crucial oils.

vi.    Empty the cream into the glass jugs and shake until the blend has cooled altogether to keep the oil and water from isolating.

vii.    So as to protect the vital oils keep clear containers in a dull spot.

viii.    Utilize the cream either in the morning or before you go to bed.

**25.    Skin toner for normal skin:**

**Ingredients:**

i.    Geranium oil- 2 drops.

ii.    Rosewater- 200ml.

iii.    Chamomile oil- 2 drops.

**Method:**

i. Place the rosewater base into a perfect glass container and include geranium and chamomile oils.

ii. Close the jug and shake the blend energetically to scatter the oil.

iii. A scattering specialist is regularly included business blends, however since this is crisply homemade we will prohibit it.

iv. Leave the blend for no less than 36 hours before shaking it again energetically and after that sifting it through a paper espresso channel to expel the bigger measure of fundamental oil.

v. Re-bottle the separated toner and recollect shaking it before use to guarantee legitimate conveyance of the blend.

**26. Skin toner for oily skin:**

**Ingredients:**

i. Rosewater- 200ml.

ii. Rose otto- 2 drops.

iii. Juniper berry- 2 drops.

**Method:**

i. Place the rosewater base into a perfect glass container and include rose otto and juniper berry.

ii. Close the jug and shake the blend energetically to scatter the oil.

iii. A scattering specialist is regularly included business blends, however since this is crisply homemade we will prohibit it.

iv.     Leave the blend for no less than 36 hours before shaking it again energetically and after that sifting it through a paper espresso channel to expel the bigger measure of fundamental oil.

v.      Re-bottle the separated toner and recollect shaking it before use to guarantee legitimate conveyance of the blend.

**27.      Skin toner for dry skin:**

**Ingredients:**

i.      Weak infusion of chamomile- 200ml.

ii.     German chamomile- 2 drops.

**Method:**

i.      Place the rosewater base into a perfect glass container and include dilute chamomile infusion and German chamomile.

ii.     Close the jug and shake the blend energetically to scatter the oil.

iii.    A scattering specialist is regularly included business blends, however since this is crisply homemade we will prohibit it.

iv.     Leave the blend for no less than 36 hours before shaking it again energetically and after that sifting it through a paper espresso channel to expel the bigger measure of fundamental oil.

v.      Re-bottle the separated toner and recollect shaking it before use to guarantee legitimate conveyance of the blend.

**28.      Bronzing caffeine body bar:**

**Ingredients:**

i.      Cocoa powder- 1 teaspoon.

ii.      Cocoa butter- 1/2 cup.

iii.      Pinch of cinnamon.

iv.      Coffee infused coconut oil- 1/2 cup.

v.      Cornstarch- 1 teaspoon.

vi.      Beeswax- 2 tablespoons.

**Method:**

i.      To begin, melt the butter beeswax and coconut oil altogether.

ii.      Expel from warmth and blend in the cocoa powder, cinnamon and cornstarch.

iii.      Empty softened butter into a mold, biscuit tin or even ice solid shape plate.

iv.      Give blend a chance to cool until solidified.

v.      Pop out the bars and store in a tin or jug.

## 29.        DIY lemon hand lotion:

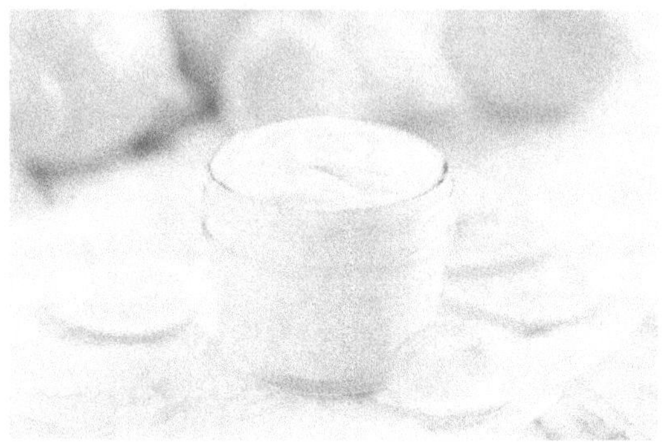

### Ingredients:

i.      Glycerin.

ii.     Lemon juice- 6 tablespoons.

iii.    Air tight container.

### Method:

The method for this cream is extremely simple. Simply, blend the fixings and spot in the holder. At that point apply to your hands and appreciate the smoothing, saturating impact.

**30.       Whipped coconut lotion:**

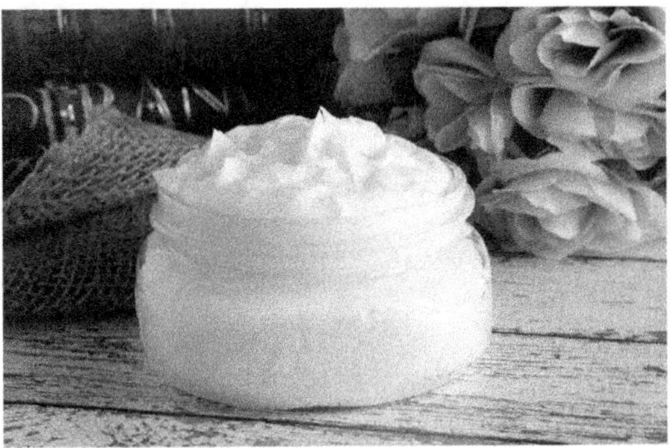

**Ingredients:**

i.      Coconut oil.

ii.     Peppermint oil.

iii.    Container with lid.

iv.     Lavender oil.

v.      Aloe vera gel.

**Method:**

i.      To start with, whip the coconut oil. It should be strong for this so stick it in the cooler for a bit in the event that it is excessively fluffy.

ii.     At that point put the oil into a dish and blend for 10 minutes with a hand blender until it gets fleecy.

iii.    At that point include a couple drops of key oil and blend in a bit of aloe vera gel. Blend well.

### 31. Calendula-aloe lotion:

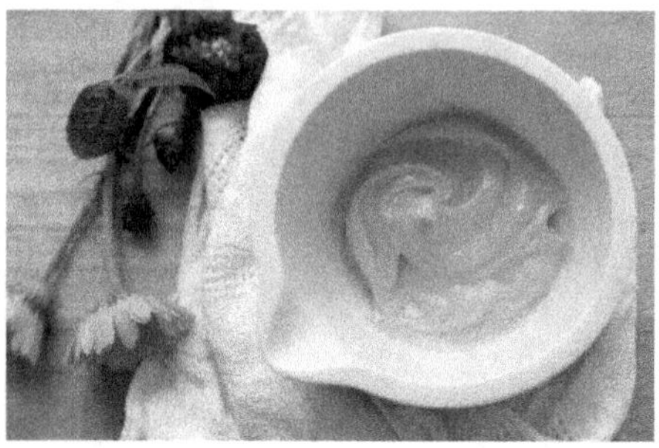

### Ingredients:

i.      Calendula oil- 6 tablespoons.

ii.      Raw honey- 1 tablespoon.

iii.      Chamomile essential oil- 20 drops.

iv.      Aloe vera- 1 tablespoon.

### Method:

i.      Empty every one of the fixings into a perfect or sterile jug and shake to combine.

ii.      Test in a discrete spot to check for bothering.

iii.      Wash the influenced zone, shake container to join fixings and delicately apply the cream.

iv.      Store in the cooler, as the cool temperature will alleviate, as well.

v.      The crude honey implies this is not appropriate for children under one year of age.

# Chapter 5 – Organic Lotions Based on Butter

Butter is one of the key ingredients used in organic lotions. They are used in lotions to maintain their consistencies as well as they add a fine texture to the lotion. These bars are based on some of the vital ingredients used to fulfill the oil demands of a dry skin; some of the recipes for butter based lotions are given below:

**32.**    **Lemon cream body butter:**

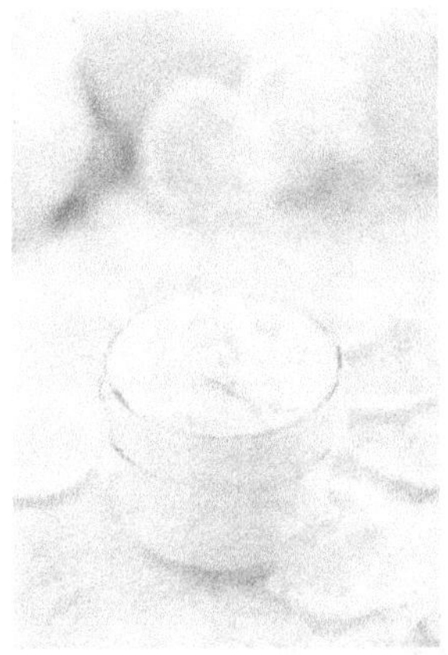

**Ingredients:**

i.      Coconut oil- 6 tablespoons.

ii.     Lemon essential oil- ¼ teaspoon.

iii.    Vitamin E oil- 4 tablespoons.

iv.     Cacao butter- 1/4 cup.

**Method:**

i.      To begin, put coconut oil and the cacao butter in a pan. Heat them till hey melt.

ii.     Afterwards, turn off the heat and include Vitamin E oil in them.

iii.    Now let it cool and solidify.

iv.     Transfer to your required container.


**33.     Vanilla bean body butter:**

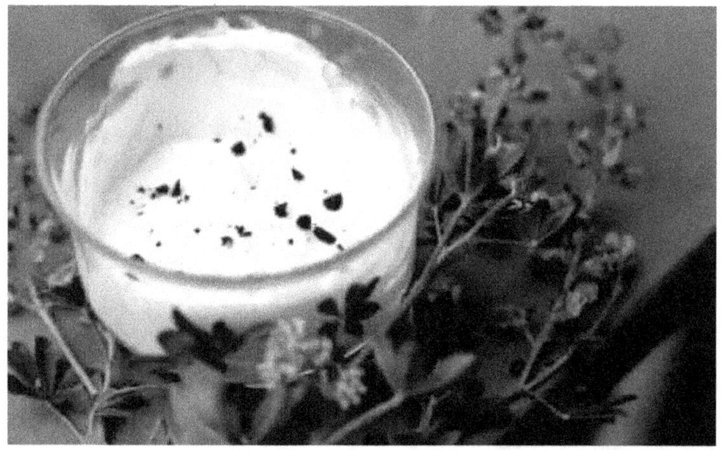

**Ingredients:**

i.      Cocoa butter- 2 cups.

ii.     Coconut oil- 1.

iii.    Vanilla beans- 2.

iv.     Sweet almond oil- 1.

**Method:**

i.      To begin, put coconut oil and cocoa butter in pan and melt. Afterwards, let it cool for some time.

ii.     Use grinder to grind the vanilla bean.

iii.    Add almond oil, ground vanilla beans in to the cooled mixture.

iv.     Now, put them in freezer and solidify them.

v.      Combine them and mix using an electric mixer to make butter like consistency.

vi.     Your cream is ready.

**34.    Coffee butter foot cream:**

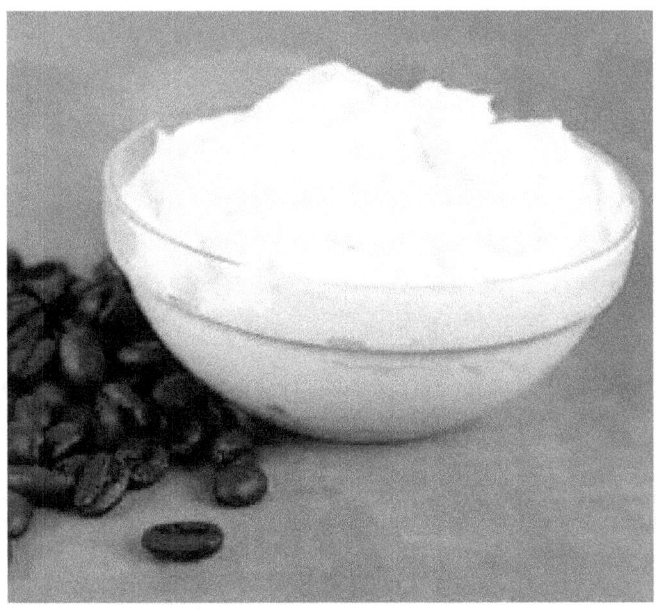

**Ingredients:**

i.      White Beeswax.

ii.     Optiphen.

iii.    Coffee Butter.

iv.     Peppermint 2nd Distillation Essential Oil.

v.      Sunflower Oil.

vi.     Dark Rich Chocolate Fragrance Oil.

vii.    Stearic Acid.

viii.   Distilled Water.

ix.     Emulsifying Wax.


**Method:**

i.      Firstly, melt all of the wax, butter and sunflower oil altogether.

ii.     Now add distilled water in a container and heat it.

iii.    Afterwards, add oil in water and blend them together.

iv.     When the temperature is appropriate, include chocolate fragrance oil, optiphen and peppermint essential oil. Combine them together.

v.      Put the lotion in jars and let them stay.

**35.**     **Anti-bacterial body butter:**

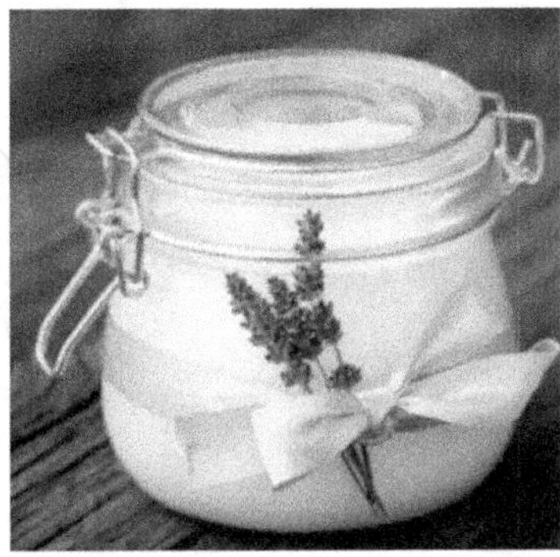

### Ingredients:

i.      Coconut oil- 1 cup.

ii.     Melrose essential oil- 30 drops.

iii.    Cocoa butter- 12 tablespoons.

iv.     Progest E.

v.      Jojoba oil- 4 tablespoons.

### Method:

i.      To begin, melt the cocoa butter.

ii.     Afterwards, add jojoba oil, coconut oil and then whisk them together.

iii.    Solidify the mixture by putting it in the freezer for a night.

iv.     Now, grind the solid and add Melrose oil and stir.

v.      Your lotion is ready.

**36.      Black raspberry vanilla body butter:**

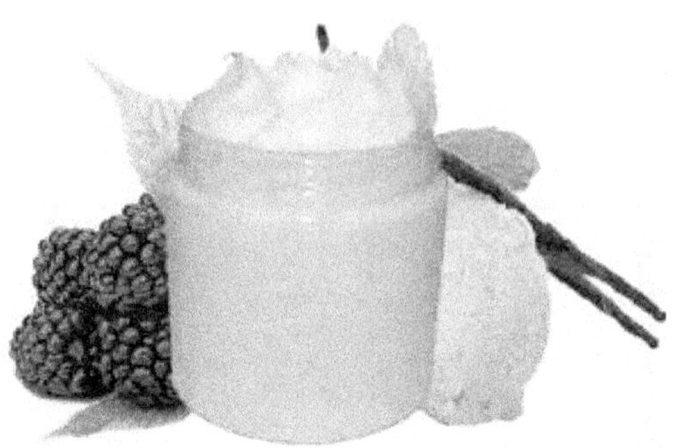

**Ingredients:**

i.      Apricot Kernel Oil.

ii.     Cocoa Butter.

iii.    Black Raspberry Vanilla Fragrance Oil.

iv.     Shea Butter.

v.      Vitamin E Oil.

vi.     Grapeseed Oil.

**Method:**

i.      Weigh out the majority of your spreads, apricot bit oil, and the grapeseed oil.

ii.     Start softening the spreads and weighed out grapeseed oil and apricot bit oil. Heat until totally liquefied.

iii. Once dissolved, expel from warmth source and include the Black Raspberry Vanilla Fragrance Oil and blend subsequent to including Vitamin E Oil.

iv. Empty the blend into a blending dish and set in cooler to cool.

v. As it cools the blend will get to be thicker. At regular intervals or something like that, utilization a hand blender, and whip the spread for a few minutes.

vi. Once the spread has set the distance and is no more runny, spoon it into your jugs and you are done.

**37.  Peppermint body butter:**

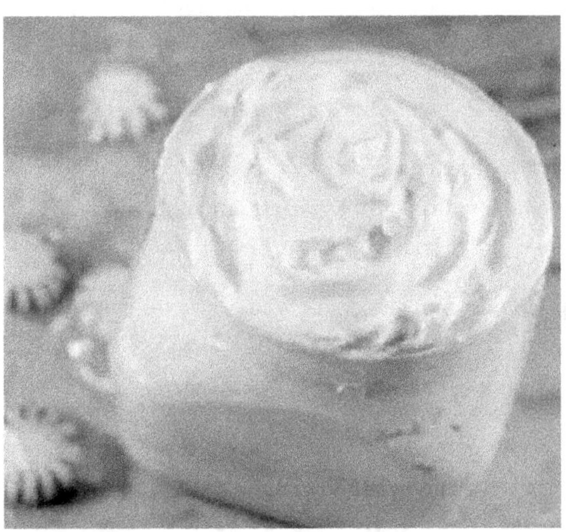

**Ingredients:**

i.      Coconut Oil.

ii.     Rubbing Alcohol.

iii.    Food coloring.

iv.     Mason Jars.

v.      Cocoa Butter.

vi.     Essential oil depending upon your choice.


**Method:**

i.      Shower a capacity holder with rubbing liquor and put aside to dry.

ii.     In a twofold kettle, melt both the coconut oil and cocoa spread. When oils are dissolved, expel from warmth and refrigerate.

iii.    Once the oils seem hazy, expel from refrigerator and utilizing a stand or hand blender whip. The oils will get smooth quick.

iv.     When oils are velvety, refrigerate for 4-6 minutes, and after that keep on whipping once more. Include fundamental oils, and whip until you get solid tops.

v.      Separate into two bowls, and shading one with the color of your choice. Utilizing a spoon or funneling sack, include a layer of butter and then a coloring exchanging until compartment is full.

**38.       Coconut rose body butter:**

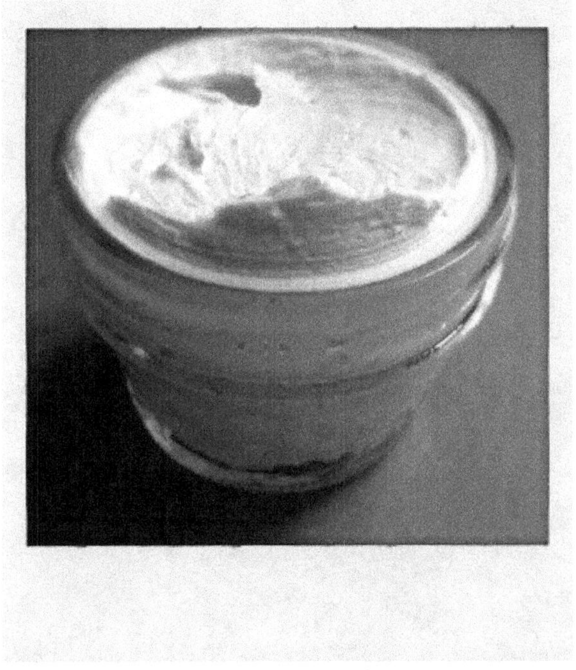

**Ingredients:**

i.      Coconut oil- 30 grams.

ii.     Jojoba oil- 5 grams.

iii.    Alkanet infused oil- 1/2 ml.

iv.     Cornstarch- 1 1/2 grams.

v.      Rose essential oil- 5 drops.

**Method:**

i.      Firstly, combine the alkanet mixed oil, jojoba oil, coconut oil, and the cornstarch in a glass dish. Heat it till the coconut oil is liquefied. Mix it once again and permit to cool to room temp.

ii.     When blend is cooled to room temp, include your key oil and stir the mixture until the mixture becomes fluffy

iii.    Place the mixture into a little container.

**39.      Rosemary mint whipped shea body butter:**

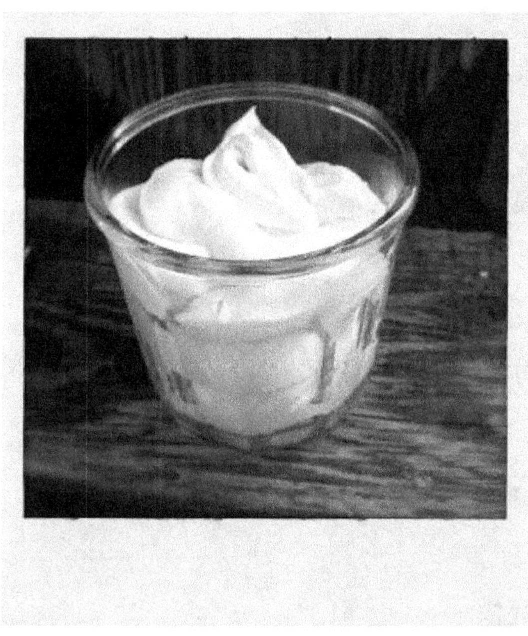

**Ingredients:**

i.      Cocoa Butter- 90 grams.

ii.     Rosemary Essential Oil- 20 drops.

iii.    Shea Butter- 180 grams.

iv.     Spearmint Essential Oil- 3 teaspoons.

v.      Kukui Nut Oil- 90 grams.


**Method:**

i.      Assemble your fixings. Cocoa margarine is truly hard and is now and again precarious to break into pieces, be cautious.

ii.     In a medium estimated glass or metal dish, apportion your Cocoa Butter.

iii.    Include your Shea Butter. Shea Butter is sufficiently delicate to be effortlessly scooped out the container.

iv.     Presently, shower in the Kukui Nut Oil.

v.      Place the blow away a dish of stewing water and permit the margarines and oil to liquefy over low warmth.

vi.     Permit the softened blend to cool at room temp for around 15 minutes and afterward exchange to your cooler for quite a while.

vii.    Mix blend with a whisk connection for around 5 minutes and spot once more into the cooler.

viii.   Watch how it is beginning to turn rich hued. Continue whisking and if fundamental come back to the cooler until blend is super frosty.

ix.   Verging on prepared, simply continue whisking. Scratch down the sides of the dish as required. This is the moment that you can include your key oils.

x.   Utilize this moisturizer within 60 days.

# Conclusion'

Individuals have been utilizing beauty items since quite a while. In this way, keeping in mind the end goal to saturate their skin, they utilize the utilization of lotions and sunscreens. These moisturizers are made commercially, as well as, a large number of individuals made the comparative items at home.

In spite of the fact that, the business creams can be solid initially, yet they have different poison chemicals, which can hamper the skin cells. Considering this issue, the significance of natively constructed items appears to be unavoidable. Along these lines, this book is intended to give productive salve formulas, which can be made at home.

This book covers various sorts of formulas to enhance the skin. To start, the formulas for hand crafted creams for oil skin are incorporated. Moreover, the formulas which are utilized to make natural moisturizers for dry skin are examined.

Notwithstanding that, the formulas for men moisturizer are expounded. Besides, the formulas which help you in making moisturizers for unbiased skin are likewise consolidated in the book. At long last, the formulas, which help in the making of spread based moisturizers are enveloped.

In this way, this book is an astonishing manual to make hand crafted moisturizers. The moisturizers made utilizing these formulas will help you in enhancing your skin. Additionally, they don't have destructive chemicals which can bring about various issues.

It is a result of the effectiveness of the custom made salves that they are utilized universally as a part of different parts of the world. In this way, keeping in mind the end goal to enhance your skin, you should begin utilizing the hand crafted salves at this moment. Further, the formulas included here will control you to start making and utilizing non-dangerous and skin cordial creams.

# FREE Bonus Reminder

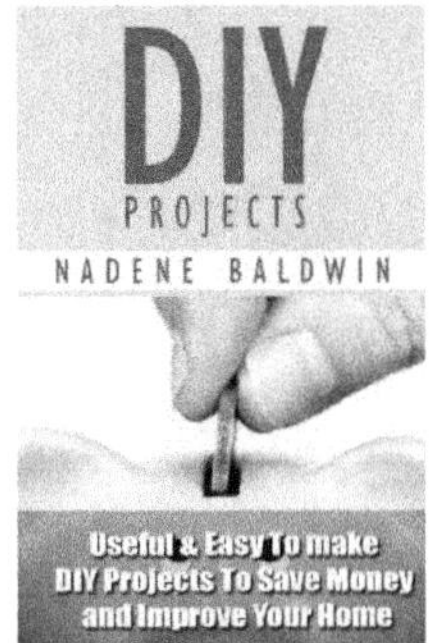

If you have not grabbed it yet, please go ahead and download your special bonus report *"DIY Projects. 13 Useful & Easy To Make DIY Projects To Save Money & Improve Your Home!"*

Simply Click the Button Below

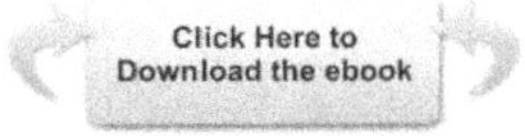


OR **Go to This Page**

**http://diyhomecraft.com/free**

## BONUS #2: More Free & Discounted Books or Products

**Do you want to receive more Free/Discounted Books or Products?**

We have a mailing list where we send out our new Books or Products when they go free or with a discount on Amazon. Click on the link below to sign up for Free & Discount Book & Product Promotions.

**=> Sign Up for Free & Discount Book & Product Promotions <=**

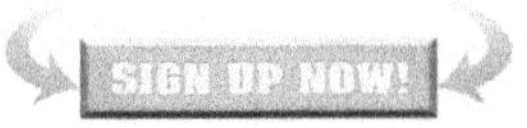


OR Go to this URL

**http://zbit.ly/1WBb1Ek**